MW01296914

Jennifer Heard

Tourette's Syndrome: Control Through Yoga Therapy

Jennifer Heard

Yoga Therapy

For the Management of
Tourette Syndrome

Jennifer Heard DNM, DHS

DEDICATION

I dedicate this book to my family: my loving husband and 3
beautiful children.

The appendix includes charts that can be photocopied or used as templates to make your own. My clients have found these very useful while working towards their specific goals. The ones included in this book are generalized to suite the public. I encourage you to produce your own customized to your unique situation. Another great option is a journal or several; to keep in handy places so that you can record feelings as they occur. This is a great way to keep track of triggers and those things that calm the nerves. After a month or so you begin to see patterns; when this happens it is easier to avoid trigger situations and to know how to handle them when they are impossible to avoid.

Personal stories have been reproduced with permission from clients and their practitioners. Names have been changed to protect identities. I want to thank everyone who has shared their personal experiences in order to help others manage their symptoms of Tourette Syndrome.

Jennifer Heard

Tourette Syndrome:

An Overview

Struggle
Compulsion
Anxiety
Fear

I move through life:
Not really

I wander through darkness:
Never fitting

I see, I feel, I am here:
But I worry
Do you see, Do you feel, Do you recognize me?

Can I be all that I want:
That you want?
Without losing who I am?

YES

Jennifer Heard

"Mom, my hands hurt" six year old Ben announces as he walks in the door from school. Ben's knuckles are inflamed, swollen and red. His mom is shocked! Over the next few days the swelling does not go down and Ben is now shaking his hands to the point that it looks as if they will fly right off his arms. "Why are you shaking your hands?", "because they hurt, shaking makes them feel better"….

Tourette syndrome is a complicated, inherited neurological disorder that often presents in early childhood. It is characterized by physical (motor) tics and phonic (vocal) tics. The symptoms are widely varied and affect people in many different ways. The tics may come and go and change over time becoming more complex as the child ages towards puberty and lessening into adulthood sometimes disappearing all together. Many patients report they are able to temporarily suppress tics but that the suppression usually results in an uncontrollable release in the near future.

Tourette Syndrome is considered to be an autosomal dominant (meaning you only need to receive the gene from one parent for expression) genetic syndrome; however the exact location has not been identified with 2 possible loci indicated in a 1992 study. There is also further debate whether the gene is maternal, paternal or both. The theory that the gene resides on the male chromosome, was developed because the incidence of Tourette's is greater among males than females. It was theorized that when a father has Tourette Syndrome he may pass it to his daughter through crossovers that occur during mitosis; whereby the gene for Tourette's crosses from the Y-chromosome onto the X-chromosome.

Location on the Y-chromosome has been dismissed in recent

years with some believing that Tourette Syndrome can be inherited from both parents giving the child two chromosomal loci which increases the intensity of expression. No further supporting research has proven or disproven these findings since the early 1990's. The general thoughts are that there are several factors at play that determine if the gene is to be expressed and where exactly the gene is located. Theories on factors that may promote expression include childhood infection, maternal stress and wellness during pregnancy, or if the child has one or two genes.

Some believe that Tourette Syndrome is a spectrum disorder which may be inherited with other disorders making it that much harder to pinpoint. These same groups believe that Tourette's and Attention Deficit Hyperactivity Disorder (ADHD) are linked one indicating the other with several manifestations of the two existing. This is highly controversial as there are many people that suffer one without the other. Finally there is an idea that Tourette's may occur on different genes in different families. If this is the case then surely Tourette Syndrome would be considered more of a situational disorder. Further research needs to be done to discover the exact cause, occurrence or expression rate and genetic patterns; as the incidence of Tourette's expression rises this research will be conducted. For now we must learn the tools available to manage Tourette's that do not exacerbate the situation or cause further dis-ease within the body in the present moment or for the long run.

Although considered genetic it is possible to carry the marker for Tourette's and never have it show up. Or maybe a person will have a very brief encounter. If they do not know Tourette's runs in the family they will chalk it up to bad nerves. This is sometimes referred to as situational Tourette Syndrome.

Let us look at the case of Ben and Alex; brothers with a father who has Tourette's; if it is a Y-chromosome dominant gene then both boys have it. Ben, the older boy, has shown symptoms since the age of 4. For the most part Ben is a nervous person. Alex is extremely laid back and has never exhibited any signs, except once. For about 3 months during a trying family ordeal Alex rolled his eyes, chewed on his shirt and made an audible squeak under his breath. These tics were constant for approximately 3 to 4 months. The tics left as suddenly as they appeared and have not recurred in the last 4 years. Why?

Alex is a social, well-adjusted child that is involved in many activities and gets good grades. Ask anyone who knows him and they will tell you he "goes with the flow". His brother is quite the opposite. Ben is a high achieving, introvert who excels academically and puts pressure on himself. As a child he was uncoordinated and did not put his physical energy to good use. We can go on about the differences of their childhoods as the boys are 5 years apart. When Alex's tics arose he already had all the tools he needed to manage them. Ben did not. His family had just moved, he was starting a new school, without friends and a baby brother on the way. Ben had no idea what stress was until it hit full on!

Tourette's itself does not impair one's mental capacities or their ability to learn however it often has comorbid conditions that cause more problems than the syndrome itself. TS can go hand in hand with other syndromes; such as Obsessive Compulsive Disorder (OCD), Attention Deficit Disorder (ADD), Attention Deficit Hyperactive Disorder (ADHD), general anxiety and learning disabilities. It is interesting to note here that studies show yoga to be a great way to help manage all of these syndromes as well.

Sufferers of Tourette's experience symptoms in the form of tics which are repetitive, non-rhythmic movements or sounds that are felt as a need for release. As in the case of a sneeze, the nose tickles or itches causing a sneeze; this is the case with Tourette's where some un-comfort or misfire by the nervous system produces the need to shrug the shoulders, or blink an eye etc.

Motor tics are movement-based and can be classified as either simple or complex. Simple tics involve only one muscle group and may often go unnoticed. These may include eye twitches, rolling of the eyes, shrugging of the shoulders, a slight "chuff" sound made under the breath, etc. Complex tics may involve 2 or more movements and sometimes can also incorporate vocal tics. Kicking legs, flailing arms, uttering sentences are some examples.

Sounds produced by the throat, mouth or nose are considered phonic tics; while Coprolalia, is the utterance of words and obscenities. This rare form of TS is what the disorder has become known for. When in fact it is present in a small minority of people that suffer with Tourette's.

All types of tics can come and go often without rhyme or reason; however some people report that tics are worsened by stress and anxiety levels. Some adults that thought their symptoms had vanished may experience short bursts during times of high stress: which can further exacerbate their stress levels.

Often Tourette's goes undiagnosed but it is estimated that 0.4% to 3.8% of children ages 5 to 18 have Tourette's. Children will often "grow out of it" making Tourette's Syndrome into adulthood rare; those adults that do suffer often feel isolated and ashamed. Many times feeling the need to "hide" outbursts or to suppress them until they are able to release in private.

In most cases Tourette's Syndrome is not treated; when it is, it is controlled by powerful pharmaceuticals that cause more problems than they fix.

I believe the combination of healthy diet and yoga practice can reduce the need for medicated control of Tourette's Syndrome leading to a healthier, happier life.

Let's take a step back and see if we can understand TS from a physical perspective.

The Nervous System

The nervous system (NS) controls every aspect of what we do; it is the body's headquarters. Made up of the Central and the Peripheral Nervous System, nerve fibers cover the entire body. In fact if we were to remove all others parts of the body so that we only saw nervous fibers we would be able to identify every aspect of the body, the size, shape and gender would all be revealed!

Here is a brief overview of the Nervous system:

- *Central Nervous System* (CNS) is made up of the brain and spinal cord.

- *Peripheral Nervous System* (PNS) is made up of nerves and nerve bundle that connect the CNS to every part of the body.

- *Sensory Division* transmits physical stimuli such as touch, sound and light to the brain.

- *Motor Division* transmits signals to muscles and glands.

- *Somatic Nervous System* sends signals to the skin, joints and muscles and governs voluntary movements

- *Autonomic Nervous System* sends signals to smooth muscles, cardiac muscles and glands; the ANS is involuntary. I can be divided in to 2 systems SNS and PNS.

- *Sympathetic Nervous System (SNS)* is generally responsible for action as in the fight-or-flight response maintaining bodily function during action and/or stress. The SNS takes care of the quick response always at the ready. It works in complementary opposition to the PNS.

- *Parasympathetic Nervous System (PNS)* is responsible for the "rest and digest" function of the body. It is slow to react and does most of its work while we are sleeping.

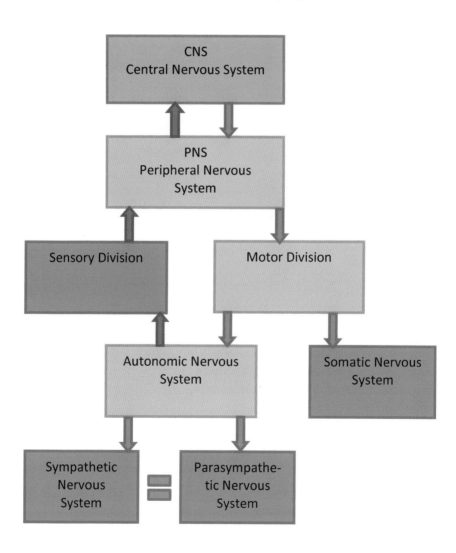

The above diagram is an extremely simplified overview of how the nervous system works. In reality the PNS is extremely complicated with every division working on its own and in conjunction with the others to allow the body to function optimally. For the most part we do not need to know what each system does just that it works and that each system needs a bit of the others to maintain a healthy body and mind.

The body moves by way of nervous impulse. An electric current runs through pathways of nerve fibers to send signals that tell us to lift the fork, maneuver a portion of pasta onto the fork and then bring it to our lips. The nervous system never rests; if it did we would die. Breath, heartbeat, brain activity are all reliant on this one system. When it fails we call it a syndrome. Tourette's falls under this classification.

The misfire of nervous fiber sends signals that we did not ask for; twitches, sounds, movements otherwise known as tics. For the most part the NS acts unconsciously, we can tell our hands to move. Often though we are moving before we have the chance to verbally say "move"!

Try it: tell your hand to lift away from this book. I bet the hand moved before you had a chance to finish saying the words? This is because as you read the instruction to move the hand your NS reacted before the mouth could formulate the words. Ever notice that you can read faster in your mind than out loud? This is because it is a direct route. The eyes (made up of all nerves) are directly connected to the brain. To read silently it is a two-step process to read aloud it is four steps. (1) eyes see the writing (2) brain analyses the words (3) brain tells mouth (vocal cords & tongue) to formulate the words (4) voice is emitted.

The nervous system is under a lot of pressure everything we encounter, every reaction has to come via this organization of fibers. Today we are constantly connected to every possible source of stress out there. When was the last time you turned off your phone, laptop, tablet, etc.? Have you been unreachable in the last 10 years? Not many of us have! This is one reason we are seeing an increase in nervous disorders. There is no down time for the body to regulate. If Tourette Syndrome is truly a cause and effect syndrome then we are causing it to occur more frequently.

Ben's swollen knuckles had been bothering him for a couple weeks, he was shaking his hands to ease the pain. The family doctor suspected juvenile arthritis was the cause of Ben's inflamed and swollen knuckles so he was sent to a pediatric specialist. At the age of 8 Ben was formally diagnosed with Tourette's Syndrome, during the pediatric interview the father was also diagnosed. Instead of juvenile arthritis, it was the shaking that had been causing the pain and inflammation.

During the interview the pediatrician noticed small motor ticks that Ben's father was exhibiting. He had a reason for every one; eye blinking because he wore contacts (yes he did it before contacts but that was because of poor eyesight), throat clearing was due to allergies... there are more but I'm sure you get the point. Tourette's Syndrome is easily overlooked or misdiagnosed in well adjusted children.

Over a few short months the symptoms of Tourette's became more noticeable the pediatrician wanted to begin pharmaceutical control. Before this could happen A LOT of questions needed to be answered.

The drugs currently being used for treatment cause a large number of adverse side effects that can reduce quality of life, cause physical damage to major organs, lead to alternate syndromes which themselves are then medicated, further complicating things.

What are the main drugs for TS control?

There are many different drugs used in the treatment of Tourette's, in most cases it is a case of trial and error. People often go through several different ones before finding the one that works best for their unique case. Of course other factors come into play that may require drugs of a different class. As in cases where ADHD, OCD and other complications are also involved.

Some of the more common pharmaceuticals used in the control of Tourette's include: *Risperidone, Ziprasidone Haloperidol, Pimozide, Fluphenazine, Clonidine, Guanfacine*

Each of these pharmaceutical drugs carries side effects that range in severity which may include any or all of the following plus others that are occur less frequently:

- They can cause abnormally high levels of prolactin a hormone responsible for breast enlargement and lactation.

- Headache, dizziness

- Respiratory disorders

- Digestive disorders including: nausea, vomiting, diarrhoea, constipation, flatulence gastritis, gastroesophageal reflux

- Central nervous system disorders including: Tremor, Dystonia, Akathisia, Parkinsonism, Spasmodic movement, vertigo (funny how these drugs are used to control motor tics but it can also cause several nervous system disorders)

- Abnormal vision

- Weight gain leading to obesity or weight loss leading to anorexic symptoms

- Rash, allergic dermatitis, psoriasis, skin irritation

- Anxiety, panic attacks

- Palpitation, chest pain, increased heart rate, tachycardia

- Joint stiffness, muscle cramps

- Pain in extremity

- Urinary incontinence

- Acne

- Restless legs syndrome

- Erectile dysfunction

Are you scared yet? I was while researching these side effects for the use of these drugs on my son. Long term use of any one of these drugs can lead to liver and/or kidney failure, chronic depression, heart attack... Careful consideration is advised when considering a course of pharmaceuticals.

What harm can come from not medicating?

When TS is not linked to other syndromes that are life threatening (severe depression, schizophrenia etc. which require close attention and may *need* to be managed with pharmaceuticals) no physical harm can come from refusing medications.

In the cases of severe motor or verbal tics social problems may develop, therefor we need other methods for controlling these tics.

Can TS be controlled in any other fashion?

What good can come from not medicating?

Yes Tourette's Syndrome can be controlled in different ways! The next few chapters will discuss some natural alternatives to pharmaceutical drugs that do not place undue stress on the body. As unique beings success will vary between people. The following is a guideline, whenever possible it is advised to seek medical attention to help oversee the course of action. Doctors of Natural Medicine, Naturopaths, Holistic Nutritionists, Yoga Therapists, Chiropractors and Counsellors are great people to talk to. By giving people choice in therapy they can reduce the need for pharmaceutical control of ticks associated with Tourette's.

How does Stress Affect Tourette's?

When confronted with danger, or a "stressor," we respond with a "fight or flight" response in the body. It is this response to stress that kept the cavemen alive and allowed the evolution of the human species. Stress, under normal circumstances, protects us from danger and brings awareness to our surroundings in order for us to react. Just the idea of stress can cause anxiety in some people; for others it is just a word. A recent study showed that the way we react to the idea of stress has more impact on our health then the stress itself. In fact stress is not a bad thing; it is our reactions that are. Yoga and mindfulness can change the way you perceive stress removing anxiety and replacing it with something better: HEALTH!

When the body perceives a stressor multiple hormones are released to help the body handle the stressor. The neurotransmitter acetylcholine stimulates the body to release norepinephrine (noradrenaline) which signals that all nervous tissue is stimulated and called to attention. Let's look closely at Hydrocortisone: a steroid hormone released in response to stress to increase blood sugar, and aid in the metabolism of carbohydrates, fats, and proteins so that the body is ready to "fight" or "run".

Cortisol also suppresses the immune system and decreases bone formation. In small amounts, under the right circumstances, this is good as it allows the body to be "at attention" for any action needed. However long term stress causes too much cortisol to be released, too often; which can lead to a malnourished skeletal system and high blood sugar levels. The malnourished body cannot perform optimally, when you add the genetic makeup for Tourette's Syndrome to this mix the nervous system goes into overload and tics become worse. The stress of having tics and trying to hide it result in more stress and we end up in a vicious cycle.

Now the good news: stress also stimulates the release of the hormone oxytocin (the "cuddle" hormone). When we feel good, have positive social interactions, experience love and physical contact oxytocin is also released. Recent studies have shown that oxytocin is a "healing" hormone, it has the ability to modulate inflammation and promote healing, one the few hormones that can bind directly to heart tissue promoting repair. This hormone has also been shown to increase empathy thereby increasing one's ability to trust and reduces fear. In very recent years many studies have been done and are still going on promoting the benefits of oxytocin in the human body.

Stress can be defined as "the body's response to a demand for change" according to Hans Selye, 1936. Change is not bad! In fact change has the ability to produce good, even great, outcomes. Remember here that the body has the same physical reaction to "good" and "bad" stress. Take the "stress" of stepping onto a stage how you react mentally depends on the crowd's response, how you react physically is chemical; the same no matter how the audience reacts. When you are applauded you beam, excited, when the applause are few to none you become sick feeling. The difference is entirely within the mind; not the body. By learning how to harness the "good" feeling (oxytocin response) we can change the mental reaction to a positive one whenever we want! In both of the above instances the same hormones and neurotransmitters are released. So every time you feel "stress" you have the opportunity to experience good instead of bad. How?

Let me provide a personal experience here. I used to dance (from 4 to 18). I was also extremely shy, I was the girl at the back of the class that did NOT speak, not ever! People terrified me; but wow did I love to dance! With dancing come recitals, in the case of my dance studio, very large productions. The feeling of being onstage was exhilarating, if the performance was not great I learned from it and practiced more, tried harder so that the next time was better. I took the terror and stress of being in front of people and used it to feel wonderful. This was a good stress, it taught me that in the face of fear I can move forward and improve myself. I'm sure you can relate with a similar type of experience! So how do we take this knowledge into other situations? Into places where the stress is "bad" and change it to "good"?

As this is a book about Yoga Therapy let us come back to that! Yoga provides us the tools to acknowledge a stressor and our reactions to it without judgment. By training the mind we can learn to examine an experience to our benefit, turning it around, mulling it over and changing the outcome. I could have shrunk in the face of fear, when I fell onstage, I could have done what I always did and shrink into the background. Instead I let the love of movement give me the strength to try again to look at why I fell not the fact that I fell. By asking why; I could change my stance and provide myself better balance to execute the move in a more graceful manner.

We will keep coming back to the question of "How?" throughout this book when we look at breath, meditation and movement.

The importance of stress management cannot be said enough! The foods we eat, the exercise we get, the air we breathe all contribute to managing, increasing, decreasing and changing this stress response.

As breath is the primary link of the mind and body bringing awareness to the breath ultimately brings awareness to the mind. This awareness can bring an understanding and a release of stress. While practicing pranayama (breathing techniques) we can use imagery to picture the stress leaving the body through the exhale and see good feelings filling up the body through the inhale.

During times of stress taking a minute to become aware of breathing will help calm the mind and slow down a racing heart. Giving you a chance to bring the body into awareness, and bring more control to the nervous system, slowing down stimulation.

Regular practice of yoga and pranayama trains the body to better handle life's stressors. Asana (yoga pose) releases tight muscles with controlled movement. When looking at a particular pose there are 3 key segments, the movements into the pose, holding the pose and then the movement out of the pose. Each of these elements contributes in a positive way to the release of stress from any given muscle group. The movement into & out of a pose strengthens muscles, uses nervous energy and brings awareness to particular muscle groups. Holding a pose for any length of time (even just a second) allows that muscle group to lengthen, strengthen, relax and oxygenate.

Yoga Therapy

Yoga, meditation and breath technique, when used correctly, can reduce the occurrence/frequency of misfires by the central nervous system. The regular practice of yoga will strengthen the small muscles which help support the body. Meditation eases the mind, brings focus and teaches control of the body. Breath technique ensures proper oxygenation of the small & large muscle groups. The average person breathes too shallow, when you add anxiety associated with Tourette's to this shallow breathing large muscles become asphyxiated increasing the probability of nervous tissue misfire.

Ben was having a really bad day, tics were out of control, as a last resource his mother put him in child's pose and massaged his back as she brought focus to his breathing. After 5 minutes Ben stopped twitching, his breath had relaxed, became smoother than normal. For the next 3 days, Ben did not tick. So started his journey through yoga and breath work.

What is Yoga Therapy? How can it help manage Tourette Syndrome?

Therapy means to remove or treat dis-ease through any means possible.

In order to remove dis-ease we must find a balance between body and mind, as the mind reacts to what the body perceives. Illness, stress, pain all derive from some imbalance within the body created by the things that we do or don't do, the things we eat and on our mental outlook.

A simple example; consider someone who is lactose intolerant. They may develop stomach upset, intestinal pain and cramping, diarrhea, gas and bloating by eating a single portion of cheese or drinking a glass of milk. It is easy to say "don't consume dairy products" because we know what the cause is. However when it comes to something like Tourette's Syndrome we know the cause of tics, but we need to find the triggers. In this case it is not so easy to say don't eat that. This is where Yoga Therapy comes into play.

Yoga is a word meaning "to join", "to attach"… it aims to bring together the body, mind and spirit through physical practice, breath technique, nutrition and spiritual awareness.

Yoga itself is a therapy. It has been adopted in the West as exercise because of the many benefits regular practice has on our physical appearance. General group yoga does not take into consideration the individual as yoga was originally intended. The ancient yogis would feel an imbalance in their body and then move into a pose (asana) to relieve that imbalance. Through these movements dis-ease was removed bringing the practitioner closer to bliss. (Important to note that the ancient yogis had very strict diets, they only consumed wholesome, natural, vegetarian foods) Through scientific research we can now use asanas to bring about healing. A forward bend removes pressure off of the lower back, therefor regular practice of stretching the spine will remove back pain. Chest opening asana gives the lungs greater space to expand which relieves symptoms of asthma, making breathing easier. Every asana has health benefits, the experienced yogi can help you find the correct ones for your body type.

Listening to our body includes what we ingest in the form of nutrients. Yoga teaches us to feel, to use our breath to become aware of all areas of the body. To do this effectively we must feed the body whole foods in order for it to heal, and grow strong.

There are many different styles of yoga under the Hatha umbrella; finding the right one for you may take some time and patience. Once you have found a style that is enjoyable it is also encouraged to do those that are not so much! Each style has something to offer its practitioners. The key to balance is on a bad day do what you love, on a good day do what you hate!

Myself: I love flow style classes; where I can get lost in the sequence and just move growing stronger, longer and more relaxed with each breath. On a bad day this is my savior. On the down side I have injuries; I know that I need yin yoga to take pressure off of my back and right hip. I know that I need deep stretching into my hips and lower back and this is what keeps me pain free. Even with all this knowledge I hate it! I struggle with yin so when I feel good and am strong mentally I head to a yin class knowing full well that I will be in pain for 90 minutes, that my head will be screaming to run as fast as possible from that room! However I also know that 90 minutes of pain and mental anguish will keep me feeling great for an entire month making my lovable classes that much more enjoyable, making daily life so much easier.

I encourage all of my patients to try as many yoga classes as they can in a week to find a good fit. If just starting out and have never tried yoga before once you find a class that you *don't hate* stick with it for a while before attempting others.

Jennifer Heard

Pranayama:

Breath Techniques

I am because I breathe
I breathe because I am

Let the breath be the sun to warm when I am cold
Let the breath be the breeze to cool when I am hot.

If the breath is the moon that guides me through the quite,
Then sun is the breath that moves me through passion.

I breathe because I am
I am because I breathe.

Jennifer Heard

Pranayama and How to Use it

Pranayama is the Sanskrit word for breathing. Broken down "prana" means life force, or breath, "ayama" means to extend or draw out; therefor "pranayama" literally means to extend the breath, to extend the life force. By extending the breath and increasing life force illness and disease can be healed. When calming breath techniques are employed 3 or more times a week, the severity of tics associated with Tourette's Syndrome is reduced.

Yoga teaches many types of breathing that can be used to control the body. The breath can bring peace and relaxation, it can focus attention, cool the body or heat it up, breath can provide a jolt of energy similar to that of caffeine without the side effects! When combined with visualization; breath can be directed to an area of unease in the body to help that area heal.

"Belly Breath" is the body's natural rhythm for the exchange of vital gases within our lungs, brought about by the movement of the diaphragm which moves the rib cage allowing for a decrease of pressure within the lungs. This pressure decrease allows the atmosphere to push air into the lungs without any work from us!

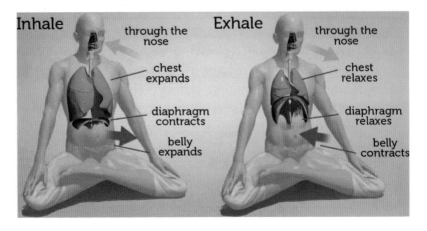

Diagram reproduced with permission from
http://www.saagara.com/learning-center

So why do we choose not to use this great tool?

The answer is both simple and complex. The simple truth is that we have become slaves to stress. "Chest breath" is a fight or flight response to a danger sign. When the body thinks danger the breath becomes shorter to allow for quicker oxygenation of the large muscle groups in preparation to fight or flee. As people, with a lot on our plates, we are in constant fight or flight mode. Basically we have forgotten how to breathe under normal circumstances. The best way to understand is to watch a baby! Notice when the baby is at rest, happy or playful the tummy moves up and down. Then, when the baby cries the breath becomes short and the chest moves up/down, she may even begin to cough and hiccup. This is our primal response; natural breath comes from the belly, stress breath from the chest.

Chest breathing, also known as, accessory breathing uses the muscles of the chest, neck and back, which are all inefficient in the act of breathing when compared to the diaphragm. The inefficiency arises from the fact that these muscles do not originate at the diaphragm therefore they do not provide enough leverage on the rib cage. A result of this inefficient breathing technique is chronic neck and shoulder pain. The shortness of the resulting breath can lead to anxiety and stress. Use of "belly breath" allows all of this tension to be relieved. By using the diaphragm for its intended purpose our breath becomes longer, without force, and our body has a better exchange of gasses; more oxygen brought in and more waste gasses removed.

Why does TS present itself in school age children? It is this breath response to stress. For the first time in their lives they are presented with a major stressor; *school.* The amount of stress a child feels is no different than that of an adult. It is only perspective. Their stress is no less than yours just because they are younger. The small body of a child is more susceptible to the side effects of long term chest breathing. They have been use to the ultimate level of oxygenation and suddenly only the large muscles are getting what they need. This rapid exchange of gases only allows for surface exchange with large muscles (the ones responsible for fight or flight). The small muscles become asphyxiated; you combine this with a genetic marker for TS and presto!

How to do the "Belly Breath"

Sit cross legged, shoulders down and back, spine straight; now take notice of your breath, do not judge, just be aware. Where is the breath; chest or belly? Is it short or long? Are you nostril or mouth breathing?

With awareness place your hands over the belly.

On an inhale through the nose expand the belly, feel your hands rise.

On the exhale, through the nose, pull the navel into the spine to release the breath.

Complete 10 rounds, then come back to simple awareness. Take note of how you feel; do you feel lighter? More calm? Is the breath deeper?

(if it is more comfortable for you, you can do this lying on your back)

Complete 10 breaths at least once a day for 2 weeks each time noting how you feel.

The belly breath is used for every other breathing exercise.

Make friends with it and it may be the only breath you need!

When ticks are at their worst the body needs a mechanism to

slow down. There are several useful breathing techniques that

can provide this downshifting of the nervous system.

The following breathing exercises are arranged in order of simplicity beginning with the easiest.

Mindful Breathing

When my son was small he would call this the *Snails Breath.*

Sit in a comfortable position with the spine tall, ensure that the head is positioned on top of the neck squarely so that your ears align with your shoulders and the shoulders align with the hips. If this is hard or uncomfortable place a pillow or block just under the hips to release the lower back. With your hands placed gently in your lap close your eyes and allow your body to breath naturally for several breaths.

Take a moment to notice if the breath originated in the chest? In the stomach? Somewhere between? Was it fast, slow, inconsistent?

Now, with intention breathe deeply in through your nose, allowing the belly to expand, then release through the nose with careful deliberation. Place one hand on the stomach and one on your chest. Again breathe in through the nose and out through the nose feeling the body expand and collapse with the breath. Focus your attention so that the breath moves the stomach out on an inhale and in on the exhale. Your chest should stay still as the breath moves through the diaphragm. Be patient with yourself, this may take some practice!

Once you can feel the breath moving through the diaphragm begin to even out the inhale and exhale. Slowing down and creating length through the breath. To stay focused it is helpful to count the breath. You may wish to count "1 inhale, 2 exhale, 3 inhale, 4 exhale..." up to 10 and then back down again.

Stay here for as long as you are comfortable with. To end the session take a deep inhale through the nose and expel it quickly through an open mouth, repeat twice more for three oral exhales.

Begin with a 5 minute set twice daily working your way up to 30 minutes once a day over a month.

The more often this is practiced the greater the benefits. Take your time; in the first session just be the observer. Watching where your breath originates, how it travels through the body. The next time you sit down add on the next step: moving the breath into the stomach to be pushed and pulled by the diaphragm. Keep adding on over time until you no longer have to think about moving the breath from the chest to the stomach. It will become a part of you. You will begin to notice that you are belly breathing most of the day. You may even notice less anxiety, less symptoms of TS. If this breath is enough for you to calm the nervous system then stay here. There is no law that says you have to move on!

Left Nostril Breathing

The ancient yogis believed that there are 3 lines of energy that run through the body: the Sushumna, Ida and Pingala. The Sushumna is the central line that connects the 7 chakras. Pingala is associated with solar energy, this line of energy begins in the right nostril. By breathing exclusively through the right nostril you create hot energy within the body. In the case of Tourette's Syndrome we are not interested in this heating activity as it can stimulate the body creating less control of motor ticks.

Our interest lies in the left nostril; where the Ida line of energy begins. This is associated with lunar energy, which is cool and calm. It is said the Ida controls the mental processes. By cooling down the mental energy we can calm the body and bring better control of motor ticks.

We begin in the same fashion as Mindful Breathing:

Begin sitting up straight and tall with your hands in your lap. With closed eyes watch your breath, focus it through the diaphragm so that the belly expands on the inhale and shrinks, pulls in towards the spine on the exhale. Take several breaths here until you feel secure that the breath is originating in the diaphragm.

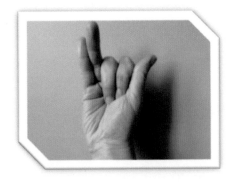

When ready raise your right hand, curl in the index and middle finger so that the thumb, ring and baby fingers are left straight. Cup the hand around the nose so that you can still breath freely. Exhale fully through both nostrils; using the extended thumb close off the right nostril, and take a slow deep inhale through the left nostril. Exhale through the left nostril this completes 1 round. Continue to breathe this way for 5 complete cycles. If counting breaths count inhale 1, exhale 2, inhale 3....until 10.

Release your hand from your nose placing gently back into your lap and breathe naturally feeling the effects for 5 breaths. Then repeat Left Nostril Breathing for 5 rounds, rest and repeat cycle. At the end of the session you should have completed 15 rounds of Left Nostril Breathing.

Over time, as you become comfortable breathing in this fashion extend the cycles by adding 2 full breaths at a time (4 half breaths: inhale, exhale, inhale, exhale) so that you breathe through the left nostril for up to 15 full breaths with 5 regular breaths between cycles.

This lead us into the last breath we will discuss here; Alternate Nostril Breathing

Purifying Breath

Alternate Nostril Breathing or "Purifying Breath" is used to centre the body and mind. By focusing your breath with intention through both nostril you bring balance to the nervous system. In 1994 a study was done showing that balance can be brought to the right and left hemispheres of the brain by alternating which nostril you breathe through. (Telles, Nagaratha & Nagendra).

This exercise creates a sense of calm alertness. The perfect balance when you need energy to get a nerve racking job done.

Sam is 15 and very nervous about a presentation he has to give in history class. The days leading up to the presentation have seen heightened activity in his motor ticks, so much so that he was asked to step out of a class to calm down. Sam's mom takes him to her yoga class the evening before the big presentation, during which they are taught Alternate Nostril Breathing. Sam begins to relax within minutes of beginning the breath. By the end of the night his ticks are no longer noticeable. What's more is that he gave a fantastic presentation that earned him his first A in history. The following day Sam and his mother sought out a private yoga instructor to teach him breathing techniques. At the time of writing this book Sam had been practicing breath and meditation for 2 years, now a senior in high school he is doing better than he ever thought possible with his grades and is looking forward to attending a good college in the fall. His motor ticks are kept in check by breath, and he no longer has to explain why his arms flail when he gets nervous.

Sam is a wonderful example of how breathing can have a very powerful effect on the body and mind.

To do this breath use the hand position from the left nostril breath:

Sitting up straight begin with 5 deep belly breaths; on the fifth inhale hold the breath for a second as you block the right nostril with your thumb of the right hand. Then exhale fully through the left nostril, with right nostril still blocked inhale through the left.

Close off the left nostril with your ring and baby finger of the right hand and exhale fully through the right, inhale, block the right and exhale left....keep alternating nostrils for 5 full rounds (5 inhales and 5 exhales through each nostril). Finish off with a final exhalation through the left nostril then place hands on your lap and breath with intention for 5 to 10 normal breaths to feel the effects.

Once you are comfortable with this breath technique do 3 rounds as above with 5 deep breaths between each round. Not everyone will have a much luck as Sam. Don't get discouraged if you don't notice progress immediately. It may take a few days of practice, remember your body is unique.

The January 2014 edition of the International Journal of Yoga published an article on the effects of alternate and unilateral nostril breathing. The study uses reaction time, heart rate and blood pressure to monitor yoga student's reaction to each type of breath exercise: Right Nostril, Left Nostril and Alternate Nostril. The study concluded that the differing types of nostril regulating breath is in tune with traditional yoga concepts of the right nostril being activating, left calming and alternating nostril balancing.

Maria went to her therapist with complex motor ticks that would leave her unable to leave the house some days. Over 6 months they changed her diet, incorporated yogic breathing (daily), meditation and a physical yoga practice 3 times a week. Her progress was slow and with many small back steps. After 6 months she had a routine down and knew what foods were potential triggers. After 1 year she went in and said she had been 2 months since her last "episode". This was the happiest anyone had ever seen her. Maria continues to keep her therapist posted on how she is doing. She believes that the breath is the key to keep complex ticks at bay. She still experiences small ticks such as eye rolls and a slight "chuff" sound now and then but she says people do not notice anymore and she is happy to be off medications.

Take your time with these exercises, there is no judgment here. Find the breath that works for you. This is just the tip of the iceberg, yoga offers many other breathing techniques that may be more beneficial to you.

I chose to include these three breaths as I have seen firsthand the benefits they offer. Your body is your temple; allow it the freedom to tell you what it needs. With time, patience and practice you will find what works and what doesn't.

The Appendix has a chart that you can use to track your breathing exercises. Use the notes section to record your thoughts and feelings as they arise. Feel free to photocopy the page or use it as a template to make your own.

Jennifer Heard

Simple Yoga Meditations

I see you world for what you are
A figment of my imagination
A string with many knots
A road with twists and turns

Moving me towards light
Begging me on an adventure

I see you thoughts
Creating a tug of war between self
As you strive for chaos
Looking for darkness. But, I choose light

Still,
Begging me on an adventure

I acknowledge you
I know you
You are I
I are we

We are adventure
We are Existence

Jennifer Heard

Meditation has been a popular topic for research over the past 2 decades. Hours of research has provided significant results proving that meditation can change neurological processes (brain function) to the benefit of the human body. One such benefit is increased concentration and self-control. The deep breathing associated with a meditative state calms the nervous system reducing symptoms of stress. The increased oxygenation of brain cells provide heightened awareness and higher brain function. We could go on as the list of benefits is endless and we continue to discover and prove them accurate as more and more research is conducted.

A study published in the Journal of Biological Psychology, September 2009 showed meditation ``to reduce or eliminate irrelevant thought processes through training of internalized attention, thought to lead to physical and mental relaxation, stress reduction, psycho-emotional stability and enhanced concentration``. This study was done to determine the effectiveness of meditation on psychiatric disorders. The study was wide spread covering a large area of mental function and the researchers involved agree that further study on individual disorders need to be performed to provide more cohesive insight on the benefits. Overall the study was successful in proving effectiveness of Meditation in disorders of affect, anxiety and those ADD related.

A brain imaging study performed at the Massachusetts General Hospital in Boston by the University of Massachusetts Medical School in Worcester studied how the brain can physically change due to a mindfulness meditation practice. The study had 16 participants meditate for 2.5 hours weekly. This study showed ``that meditation practice reduced the concentration of gray matter in the amygdala, a region associated with fear, anxiety, and stress — and that this reduction was correlated with lower stress levels`` (Results were published in Psychiatry Research: Neuroimaging: Jan. 30, 2011). As we know stress levels and the way we interpret stress has an impact on the symptoms of TS. This study lends physical proof that the brain is capable of change and we are able to make these changes by retraining the brain to think in different ways.

Over the next few pages you will find guided meditations to help ease the mind and bring about relaxation. Read over the chosen meditation a few times to make yourself familiar with the general idea before attempting to sit in meditation. Meditation is about anxiety control, if you are trying to remember what you have read the session will not be successful; in fact it may increase your anxiety level. The written words are a generalized idea of the direction to take in the mind as you guide yourself. The previous chapter looked at breathing techniques. Unless otherwise stated the only breath technique used in the following meditations is the *Belly Breath* or breathing with intention. If you have a technique that you love, use it for several rounds before beginning or at the end of the meditation.

If you prefer to listen to guided meditations I have uploaded mp3's to my website that you are welcome to listen to as you meditate. These clips are short, if you like a longer time frame begin your session with the chosen sound clip and remain in silence until you feel ready to move.

Meditating is not about creating silence in your mind, it is about learning to accept the chatter. When we meditate we use loving kindness to acknowledge the thoughts as they pass as nothing more than clouds in a bright blue sky. You see them as clouds (thoughts) but nothing more and nothing less. This is a time for you to enjoy peace. Your thoughts will be there when you are ready to examine them.

Meditation Exercise: Allowance

Give yourself permission, allowance, to be aware of your feelings. Allowance; to bring into focus that which is unclear. Allow yourself to know what you feel so that you can heal what you feel.

Close your eyes and listen: Listen to the sound of traffic outside the building, can you identify the sounds.

Bring your attention closer: outside your door, listen to the sounds of the building, your immediate surroundings.

Now even closer, hear the beat of your heart, the rush of air as it enters and leaves your body. Focus on this sound keep your attention on the breath hear it, feel it. Feel the cool calming effect it has on the body. Slow the breath down so that it is a whisper a light sound, a subtle feeling.

At this moment what do you feel? Hold this thought in your mind's eye. Examine it. Can you name it? Allow yourself to fully feel this emotion to examine the thought from all sides. Keep turning it around in your mind.

Allow the thought or emotion to slowly spin, creating lazy circles in the mind; now coming closer so that you have a clear view and slowly, slowly twisting and turning away from you until it is further, further until you can no longer see it. Allow the feelings connected with this thought to melt away. You become lighter as the sensation of the feeling drifts further and further away. A weight has been lifted off your shoulders.

Now bring your attention back to your breath. Can you notice a difference? Is it slower? More even? Watch as the breath comes and goes. Calming the body.

Hear the rush of the air in your lungs once again, getting louder, hear your heart beating, feel its pulse in your veins.

Bring that awareness outside of yourself once again. Allowing the sounds of the room, of the building to slowly come back into focus. Listen to the sounds out on the street, can you identify them? Bring with you the focus you found as you slowly open your eyes.

Meditation Exercise: Acceptance

Contentment is our natural state. We are always in pursuit of this state, however if you give yourself permission to see the happiness around you will see that you are already content. If your current state is unhappiness or stress then you must examine this state and discover the why of the current feeling/emotion. When you know the "why" you can then ask "how". How do I fix this unease? What has caused it? What is the next step I can take to remove the "un"? If the current feeling is happy, joyful ask the same questions. Why am I happy? What has caused this happiness?

When these questions are answered truthfully you can take the steps to maintain a joyful state, bringing peace to the body and mind.

Internal contentment is not the same as external contentment or happiness. When we are happy because of external circumstances it is *not* a true happiness it is still possible to have unease in the body. As Jill can attest to. Jill is a 45 year nurse in Florida: she adores her job and her life! By all external accounts she is happy. Jill and her husband both enjoy rewarding careers in the health sciences, they make enough money to go on annual holiday's, they have 2 bright boys both in their teens with great future outlook. Jill will tell you she had everything she ever wanted. This was the case when 2 years ago her Tourette's resurfaced. After 10 years of no noticeable ticks she was suddenly bombarded with complex motor ticks that left her feeling drained. Her doctor wanted to put her on pharmaceutical medications as sometimes her hand jerks would interfere with her work.

She agreed; after the third medication switch she was fed up with the side effects, the nausea, the headaches, the worsening of symptoms.... Stress was beginning to have an effect on her marriage, so her husband agreed to marriage counselling. They were lucky enough to attain the help of Leah, a counselor with a long standing mindfulness practice. She recognized that Jill may be experiencing contentment issues. From all indications she had a perfect life. Leah asked the right questions and soon discovered that Jill was not content emotionally. She felt that she did not deserve all the goodness that she was experiencing. Feelings she didn't realize she had. Jill was the confidant of a co-worker that was having life problems, as result Jill was questioning her own life internally. "why am I so lucky?" "do I deserve this?" "What if I loose all of it?" These questions and more were constantly running through her head while speaking with her friend. Hence the return of Jill's Tourette's symptoms.

Leah taught Jill to be accepting. She was encouraged to write out her internal questions, then to choose one question at a time and sit in stillness with it. By examining her negative dialogue she was able to turn it into a positive. After a session: anywhere from 5 to 30 minutes, Jill would answer her negative question with something positive. She would write out why she deserved what she had. She did not "luck out" into a rewarding career. She worked hard to put herself through school in-spite of Tourette's Syndrome and then worked her way up to the position she currently held. After 2 months of this practice the ticks began to subside. After 6 months Jill was back to herself. On check-ins Jill is content, happy on the inside. She has a daily mediation session and has recently taken up yoga classes twice a week.

True happiness can *only* come from within. This is why

answering the questions above honestly is so important.

Life is messy, by accepting your messy emotions (confusion, anxiety, depression, sadness...) and examining them you can discover who you truly are. This is when you discover true happiness, contentment within, allowing the body to heal.

After identifying your emotions or internal struggles use the *Cultivation* exercise to work with them in order to bring contentment to your body.

Cultivation

1. Define a specific attitude to cultivate (peace, tranquility, compassion, friendliness, happiness, strength, etc.) in response to your personal questions.

2. Sit comfortably, with eyes closed lengthen your breath so that you are breathing with intent; feel the silence.

3. Turn your attention to your heartbeat. Hear it, feel it. Sit here for several breaths connecting with your own natural rhythm. Say your chosen word (attitude) mentally with the next 5 inhales. Allow the exhale to take the intention and spread it like seeds in the wind. Come back to your breath and feel the silence, hear your heart.

4. Repeat step 3 for 2 to 4 more rounds always coming back to your breath in between cycles.

Practice this regularly, anytime or place with a single intention each time. Over time you will feel your awareness shift, making room for greater contentment in your life; easing pain, stress and anxiety out.

This is a generalized meditation that is wonderful for Tourette's when you know the triggers. Steve would only tick when his boss was around. The two men did not see eye to eye. Steve discovered he had Tourette's Syndrome as an adolescent; it never really bothered him, he took no actions to control it. His ticks were minor and most people never even saw it in him. In his late twenty's he was offered a promotion at work, a great opportunity to move up the company ladder. The day he met his new manager his hopes fell, they just didn't mesh. Over the next several months Steve began to really notice his TS, so did his coworkers.

It was at the suggestion of his girlfriend (Sarah, a counsellor) that Steve met with Lisa, a Yoga Therapist to whom Sarah often referred her clients. Since Steve knew that his boss was his trigger they used a similar meditation to the one above. When Steve had to meet with his boss he would take ten minutes before the meeting to cultivate patience a practice that has landed him a second promotion.

Sound Sleep Meditation

When ticks are at their height, often so is anxiety; making sleep a problem. When the body does not rest stress is increased creating a domino effect: stress – ticks – less sleep – more stress – more ticks....

Here is a simple meditation to help you sleep:

Lie on your right side, placing pillows to support the body for optimal comfort. Take 5 deep calming breaths with attention to pace and length of breath. Begin to increase the length of the exhale over the next 3 breaths. Using the *left nostril breathing technique* begin to count your breaths backwards starting at 10 going to 1. If you reach 1 take 3 deep breaths through both nostrils and begin the process again.

Allow thoughts to float past as you continue to count. Keeping a focus on the breath count keeps the mind from wandering, often a problem associated with anxiety at night.

Jennifer Heard

Nutrition

"The food you eat can be either the safest and
most powerful form of medicine or the
slowest form of poison."
— Ann Wigmore

Jennifer Heard

An Introduction to Nutrition According to Yoga

Diet, is perhaps the most important part of any health plan. There are the basic nutrients that we all need, to build and maintain the human body. Every country has their version of a food guide which states the food groups and amounts of each group that is needed for a healthy body. As far as government food guides go they each differ slightly in how foods are grouped and on which ones take precedence. As unique individuals our requirements are also unique; to some extent.

Culturally, geographically, religiously we place different rules on what we consume. The quality of our natural foods can vary depending on where it was grown and under what circumstances, if it was harvested too early or too late...

This work is not about diet; this brief section is included because any health concern is also a diet concern. If you have further questions about your diet that this work does not cover; it is highly recommended that you visit a Nutritionist or Doctor of Natural Medicine. Also there are many great books on nutrition that may suite your belief system.

To really get to know and understand how your body relates and/or reacts to the foods and beverages you ingest it is advisable to keep a detailed food and drink journal for 4 to 6 weeks. Sample journal pages are included in the Appendix.

Diet of Yoga

Ayurveda is the sister science to yoga that deals with disease, illness and nutrition. Huge textbooks have been written on the complicated subject of Ayurveda. Once understood it can answer many questions. To go into how Ayurveda can help you we need a full 200 or more page book!

It is possible however, to take a step back and look at food or nutrition, from a Patanjali point of view. If we apply the eight limbs of yoga to nutrition we can use the principles of Ayurveda in a simplified manner.

1. Yama's - Social behavior - how we relate to the world around us
2. Niyama's - Inner discipline - how we relate to ourselves
3. Asana - Physical exercise
4. Pranayama - Breath work
5. Pratyahara - Discipline of the senses
6. Dharana - Concentration
7. Dhyana - Meditation
8. Samadhi - Self realization

We have already touched on Asana, Pranayama and Dhyana (meditation) so let us now look at the Yama's. Simply put the Yama's are a set of rules that govern how we deal with or relate to the world around us; they include nonviolence, truth, abstinence and non-hoarding.

You may wonder how these virtues fit into food?

When we eat and indulge to the point of causing the body pain we are creating violence towards the body. By saying to ourselves "one more piece of cake won't hurt me" we are lying to the self and hoarding the cake making it unavailable for others to enjoy. Saying "I have enjoyed my one slice of cake" and offer the rest to another; truth and control of cravings allow us to cultivate non-violence, abstinence and non-hoarding.

Sound complicated? It's not once we get into the act of watching what and how we eat. Mindful eating allows us to see the patterns. Patters of why we eat, when we eat, what foods make us feel good emotionally and physically, those that make us feel bad or sick.

Simon came to me because his Tourette's had been out of control for 2 years during which time he had also gained 37 pounds. He had a diagnosis because it ran in his family, though he had never felt the need for medications as it had never affected his daily life. He was active as a child, on all the sports teams through adolescence, and maintained fitness into adulthood. A wonderful background! *So why now?* This question was answered when he began mindful eating.

Simon was instructed to keep a food journal, and observe feelings before and after eating. What he ate and drank, when he ate and portions. After about 4 weeks it became apparent that every time his mother called he craved sweets, homemade cookies, cakes, hot chocolate, tea with 2 teaspoons of sugar and lots of cream... If he was out and his mom called on the cellphone he would immediately head for Starbucks or any other coffee shop that had super sweet drinks and desserts. It also followed that within 2 hours after consumption of sweets Simon's tick's would start and would be bothersome for 4 to 12 hours.

Why? 3 years ago Simon's mother was diagnosed with breast cancer. She had telephoned him from her doctor's office to come be with her during the biopsy. They had one stressful year of radiation and surgery by the end of the year she was declared cancer free, but would have to undergo screenings for the next 5 years to be sure of no relapse. When Simon was a young child his grandmother (who passed away from her battle with cancer) would try to help him feel better by baking. His favorite drink as an unwell child; hot tea cooled with cream and sugar.

Mindful eating allowed bottled emotions to be recognized, acknowledged and dealt with. Simon no longer fears the phone, he has lost 42 pounds and his ticks have diminished to the point that if you did not know him you would never guess he has Tourette's.

Simon is a simple case; often it can be a number of foods or substances that trigger an outburst of ticks. Yogic eating allows us to identify the triggers so that we can learn how to manage them.

Yama - Social Behaviour

Meals are a social event, even when we dine alone! Think on it a moment...

Why do you eat what you eat?

The first time you had a sip of coffee, did you like it? or was it an acquired taste based on social pressures? How about that first beer? or glass of wine? the list can go on!

Now that you have had your first cup of coffee do you continue to drink it without a social aspect? Many people need that cup first thing in the morning; they feel the day cannot start without it. Do you fall into this category? If so why? Have you ever stopped to think about it? To understand what it is that makes that first morning cup so special that it determines your mindset for the rest of the day.

This is why nutrition is an important part of a book about yoga therapy. Taking a moment to see what foods, additives, drinks affect your symptoms of Tourette Syndrome can translate to better control.

That cup of coffee in the morning followed by one or more others throughout the day could mean the difference in severity of ticks from few to none; or lead to a day out of control.

This is perhaps the hardest part of your journey to Tourette's Syndrome management through natural means: the elimination of dietary elements.

Again I pose the question: Why do you eat what you eat?

This time look at it from a personal perspective. If you discover that coffee sets you off can you eliminate it from your diet? When it comes to your health over social acceptance can you say sure I'll go for a coffee but I'll have a cup of herbal tea instead. Can you put ego aside when your buddy's go out for a beer? Here we see Patanjali's rules of living put to use. Steps 1 and 2. Social and personal behaviors.

Coming to terms with how you relate to what you ingest is a huge step towards control and an overall better mindset. Recognizing ego for what it is and being able to say to yourself "not today" will reduce physical and mental stress in the long run.

Niyama - Inner Discipline

By eliminating all unnatural and processed foods as well as those that are known stimulants we can reset the body to discover its baseline. By finding a baseline we can add foods back into the diet to discover intolerances. Intolerance differs from an allergy in that an allergy is the body's adverse reaction to what it views as a foreign substance. Allergies cause the body to react in a defensive way to eliminate said substance from it. Food intolerance is not considered foreign; the body does not launch an attack. Instead the intolerable food causes upset as it is being digested.

A case of "the jitters" after a cup of coffee means that the body is not accepting of caffeine at this moment.

I suffered iron deficiency anemia, migraines and constipation from a young age until my mid-30's. By eliminating land animals from my diet all of these problems corrected. While my iron levels are always borderline the levels do not drop into the danger zone since the elimination of meats. I do not suggest going vegetarian. My particular constitution is happier without meat. My nutritional balance is restored and my body performs at optimal levels. A few times a month I can enjoy seafood's but one meal of chicken will disrupt digestion balance for several days. It took 6 months of trial an error to discover the line.

This is a perfect example of intolerance not allergy.

Breath

Patanjali's eight limbs of yoga include breath work. Breath or prana is life-force, we all know if we stop breathing we die. How does breath fit into nutrition? The correct question is "how does it NOT fit into nutrition"?

Proper breathing creates a favorable environment for peristalsis, muscular contractions that move along the walls of the digestive organs, to occur. Without peristalsis digestion cannot take place. As the diaphragm expands and contacts it massages the digestives organs promoting the assimilation of foods.

Proper oxygenation of the blood provides a stable transportation system to carry key nutrients from the digestive tract to areas of the body where they are needed. The blood also carries waste products to be filtered by the liver and kidneys for removal. Without adequate oxygenation the body is not able to function at top notch!

While completing the following exercises remember to breathe fully with each bite, expanding into the belly, using the diaphragm as it was meant to be used.

Exercise in Mindful Eating

What is mindful eating? On an average day we eat without thinking; breakfast, lunch, dinner and snacks. How often do you have time to stop and think about what is going into your body? Now that we have looked at the yamas and niyama's according to food it is time to meditate on the subject.

Here are 2 exercises for the next time you eat or drink:

1) Coffee Culture

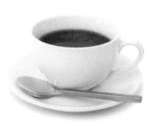

Exercise in mindful drinking; coffee not required! Use any drink you find comfort in (not alcohol)!

As you pour your cup of coffee, tea, water listen to the sound of the liquid spilling into the cup.

Feel the cup with your free hand, breathe into the feeling as the cup warms or cools with the addition of liquid.

Before you take that first sip close the eyes and hold the cup with both hands. Take 3 to 5 deep breaths feeling the weight of your chosen drink. Notice the texture of the cup, the temperature of the liquid.

Take a sip and savor it. Breathe slowly as the liquid swirls in the mouth. Mentally "chew" the liquid, feel the texture, notice the sensation it causes on your tongue, cheeks back of the throat.

As you swallow feel the warmth or coolness as it spreads down the throat. Can you sense the liquid spilling into the stomach? Follow the drinks passage from lips to mouth to throat and down into the belly.

Sit quietly with the sensations as you complete your drink.

With empty cup be thankful for the comfort the drink has provided you.

2) Mindful Meals

* Once you complete this exercise once or twice it is hard to observe an unhealthy meal.

Chose a meal to sit and watch.

Before beginning the meal take a moment to look at your plate. Notice the colours, the different textures, see the steam, smell the aroma.

As you lift the fork or spoon feel its weight. As the bite crosses your lips bring your attention here, feel the smoothness of your utensil, the different sensations of the food on the lips. Place your utensil down to chew and savor the bite.

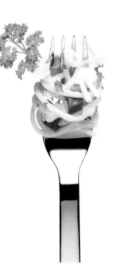

As you chew take notice, is it sweet, salty, spicy, bitter...

Be thankful for the food you are consuming.

Think about each bite for the remainder of the meal. Where did your food come from? Appreciate how it got to be on your table, all the hands that were involved in bringing you the satisfaction of this meal.

Think about how this meal is affecting your body.

Notice: did you eat as much as you normally would? I have found that the majority of people end up eating less as the stomach has a chance to tell the brain it has had enough. Weight is often gained because we eat too much at each meal. There is mind to stomach disconnect as we rush to get through the meal to move onto more pressing things. Here again we are creating stress for the self.

Continue this practice for about 2 hours after eating. Every 15 to 20 minutes stop and take a quick body scan. How are you feeling? Physically? Emotionally? Are you relaxed or stressed? Have tics increased, decreased?

After completing this exercise several times and with the aid of her food journal, Sherry found that she reacts adversely to food colourings. Within 2 hours of consuming foods with artificial colour Sherry would experience short bursts of intense motor tics. She found this to happen even when she was fully relaxed.

Sherry led a fast paced life with very little down time. Meals were grabbed on the go without attention to ingredients. She had been working with me for 3 months of yoga therapy and meditation to control her symptoms of Tourette's. When I proposed she change her diet Sherry was very hesitant. In fact it took her 2 months to finally go clean. After 1 month of healthy eating Sherry indulged in a package of red Nibs. Tics took control of her body in under 2 hours. Was it the sugar? the colour? or any of the other ingredients? For the next couple weeks she decided to watch.

Every few days Sherry ate something with artificial ingredients. With use of her food journal and mindful eating we were able to pinpoint food colouring. After so many years of unhealthy eating she never realized that food colour was a major cause of her uncontrollable tic outbursts. Sherry now enjoys a balanced diet with some of her favorite "bad" foods mingled with mostly "clean" foods of local meats and vegetables. Sherry believes that knowing is half the battle. If she chooses to indulge she knows her body will react to the colours and is prepared for this. In some cases (Nibs at the movies) she feels it is worth it!

Of course knowing is most of the battle! The ability to pinpoint trigger foods goes a long way in controlling symptoms of Tourette's. Once known the triggers can be avoided and replaced with healthy alternatives. Mindful consumption of foods and drinks speeds up the process of an elimination diet.

Let us now look at the basics. As Tourette's Syndrome is a neurological disorder there are basic nutrients that the nervous system needs to keep neurons firing appropriately: B Group, Calcium, Omega-3 and Lecithin.

Fatty Acids

Fatty acids are used by the body in the development of brain and nervous tissue. Fatty acids serve multiple functions throughout the body; proper development, cardiac health,

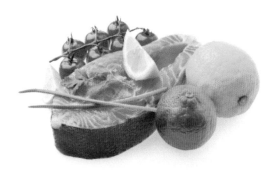

inflammation regulation, mood regulation...perhaps one of the most important in the discussion of Tourette's Syndrome is creating the myelin sheath that surrounds nervous tissue.

When the nerves are not properly coated with myelin disruptions in electrical signals occur. Research has shown that people with a thicker myelin sheath are generally less prone to anxiety and the effects of stress than those with a thinner layer.

Some fatty acids are considered non-essential because the human body if able to produce them from other key nutrients, alpha-linolenic acid and linoleic acid (Omega-3 and 6) however, are considered essential nutrients because the body is not able to create them. They must be consumed from the foods we eat. In recent years omega-3 deficiencies have been linked to developmental disorders, mental health and cognitive aging.

Good sources of essential fatty acids are: sea foods, walnuts, flaxseed, hemp, chia, sunflower and pumpkin seeds, leafy green vegetables.

B group

B-complex is a set of eight water soluble vitamins that often co-exist within foods and work synergistically together in the body. Processing foods destroys B vitamins such as when wheat is bleached. To ensure proper vitamin B intake whole foods such as whole grains, potatoes, bananas, beans and lentils should be consumed. B12 does not naturally occur in fruits and vegetables turkey and tuna are good sources. Vegans are encouraged to take a B12 supplement especially while pregnant.

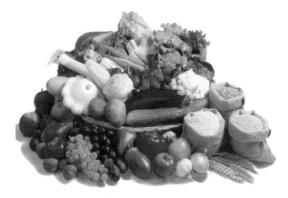

The eight vitamins that make up the B group are:

B1 – Thiamine: involved in nerve function and plays a role in the metabolism of energy from foods we eat. It is also plays a role in the production of DNA & RNA.

B2 – Riboflavin: is involved in the breakdown of fats and the production of energy in the body.

B3 – Niacin: transfers energy during the digestion of sugars, fats and alcohol and is involved in the manufacture of fats and nucleic acid in the body.

B5 – Pantothenic Acid: oxidizes carbohydrates and fatty acids and plays a role in the synthesis of hormones and neurotransmitters.

B6 – Pyridoxine: used in the breakdown of fats and amino acids and aids in the production of hemoglobin and neurotransmitters. Pyridoxine also plays an important role in the generation of glucose from non-carbohydrate substances.

B7 – Biotin: involved in the metabolism of fats, protein and carbohydrates.

B9 – Folic Acid: especially important during pregnancy and growth as it is needed for normal cell division.

B12 – Cobalamin: The body needs B12 for the production of blood cells in bone marrow, nerve sheaths and proteins

Deficiencies in B group vitamins can lead to a number of problems including: diseases of the nervous system, irregular heartbeat, heart failure, insomnia, mental confusion, muscular weakness and birth defects. If you have any concerns of deficiency consult your doctor who can order blood test to check levels.

Calcium

Calcium is an essential metal found on the periodic table with the call letters Ca and atomic number 20. Human beings cannot live without it! Cells of the body use it to communicate, when we move the muscles require calcium to contract and it is essential in the development of bones and teeth.

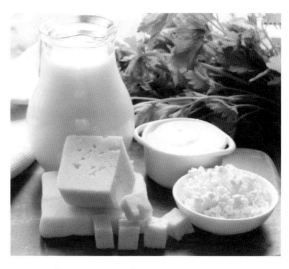

When the body is under stress and we enter flight-or-flight response mode the body excretes calcium in the urine. People that are constantly living in this state of stress are excreting calcium in large volumes. This is just one reason why the management of stress is so vital. As an important ingredient in the transmission of muscular impulse calcium must be in balance for the body to operate at optimum levels. When Tourette's is present, the individual is prone to randomized muscular impulse; the absence of calcium exacerbates the condition.

When calcium is present in such high levels on earth how do we become calcium deficient? As stated above stress is a key factor. Dietary choices also play a role here. Natural foods that contain oxalic acids, when consumed with high calcium foods, reduce the body's ability to absorb calcium; making food paring important. Avoid eating sweet potatoes, legumes, nuts, beets, rhubarb, or celery with calcium sources.

The body requires vitamin D for the absorption of calcium. When vitamin D is in short supply the regulation of body calcium is not possible. Exposing the skin to sunlight for just 30 minutes a day is enough to keep the body supply of vitamin D stocked.

Finally the consumption of acid regulating medications for heartburn prevent the absorption of calcium.

Good sources of calcium: dairy products, nuts and seeds, kale, quinoa, broccoli, dandelion leaves, and seaweeds.

Jennifer Heard

Yoga Asana

The Practice

I breathe and the airs moves from me, through me…

Eagle wings soar high above the trees waving in the breeze

Moon reflection dances on the waves: quarter, half, full and back
again

A playful dog wags and pounces atop a tall strong mountain

Whilst the cobra hissing warns off predators in the starlight

The air moves on changing, becoming, growing…

Jennifer Heard

When we say yoga asana what do we mean? Asana is one of eight limbs on the Ashtanga yoga tree as described by Patanjali. It is the physical practice, physical purification, that prepares the body and mind for mediation. Over the years Hatha yoga (the physical discipline of yoga) has become: yoga, Bikram, Vini, Flow, Power, Iyengar, Yin... to name a few! The list of new yoga disciplines continues to grow as people father or mother new versions of an ancient practice. The wonderful thing about this is that yoga has become accessible to EVERYONE! There is a style for you, if you look. Some forms barely resemble each other! The one thing they all have in common that keeps the title of yoga is that they combine breath and movement offering a union to the body and mind that we seem to have lost in day-to-day life.

When the mind and body experience trauma such as stress a disconnect can occur. Humans are very adept at ignoring and looking past instead of facing, head-on, a problem. Repeated avoidance can create walls; take for example the person that cannot find their left foot while the body is twisted. Some trauma in their life has created blocked lines of communication throughout the body. Breathing into tight areas as we move into, hold and move out of poses reignites neurons, creates new pathways thus bringing back to life these blocked lines.

Yoga heals because it brings awareness; it slows us down in our crazy lives and gives us a chance to connect. Not just to breathe, but to BREATHE for health and mental peace. For some just connecting with the breath is enough. This too is yoga! If you do nothing else but truly connect with your breath then you are doing yoga perfectly. We are not perfect creatures, if we were, you would not be reading this book! Yoga asana is a way to move the body closer to your version of ideal. By performing poses you are training the body to move in a new way. With attention paid to correct alignment we move the body closer to its natural state.

If the body has a natural state; why do we have to move towards it? Why are we not just there? Good questions! The human body was built to move. It was not built to sit all day hunched over a computer, or built to make repetitive movements for 8 hours straight as what occurs when you work a production line. Asana provides the body a way to counter balance these unnatural positions. By mimicking nature we bring in the qualities of nature. A tree is strong and stable yet moves with the wind. By grounding down through the feet in Tree Pose we create roots to the earth that provide stability. We use opposing actions in the legs to create rooted balance, the trunk of a tree. As our lungs fill and deflate the upper body moves with the force of the breath as upper branches and leaves in a breeze. We can break down every pose in this way! For now let us look at those that create a sense of calm in the body to help relieve stress.

- Poses for anxiety and stress:
- Bhujangasana (Cobra Pose
- Matsyasana (Fish Pose)
- Setu Bandha Sarvangasana (Bridge Pose),
- Salamba Sarvangasana (Supported Shoulderstand)
- Viparita Karani (Legs-up-the-Wall Pose)

It is important to remember that all yoga asana (poses) provide benefits and can help to calm heightened states. A generalization of asana classification shows us that:

Sitting and standing twists help to alleviate emotional tension.

Forward folds help to calm and ground emotions.

Back bends open the heart to release negative emotions and invite in joy.

Every yoga session should aim at balancing these characteristics to help bring balance to the mind and body. All of these ideals are incorporated into every style of yoga. So which style is best for you? The best way to find which type of yoga will most benefit you; is to attend a few classes and see which ones provide a sense of relief. There is no magic plan that tells you what will heal. I usually recommend a combination of several styles to get the greatest benefits.

Michael needs to move. He was told that yoga would help to calm his symptoms of Tourette's so he joined a restorative class. With tons of calming asana and supported postures he thought it was just what he needed. He was very wrong! Michael has a desk job where he sits for 6 to 8 hours a day. At the end of this he is wound tight and his nerves are on edge, misfiring from lack of stimuli and stress.

After making diet and other lifestyle changes I told him to seek out a power yoga class to support our one-on-one sessions. Four weeks later Michael cannot believe the difference. His ticks have slowed down and he has more constructive energy. Michael needed a release in the form of movement. The faster pace and physical demands of a power class gave his nerves a chance to fire with purpose. Michael is stronger and calmer as a result of power yoga.

Michael's story shows us that ``therapy`` was not what he

needed in this time and space. His body was misfiring from lack of exercise. Power Yoga provides the perfect balance for Tourette`s sufferers as a practice that provides the body what it needs in the form of physical exhaustion and the mind what it needs in the form of breath and relaxation.

It is important to keep this in mind when searching out a yoga practice. Most will benefit best from a combination practice of movement based and restoration based. Depending on your daily physical and mental demands each person needs stability in specific areas. This guide aims to provide an insight into how yoga, in all its incarnations, can help provide relief of the symptoms of Tourette`s Syndrome.   Yoga is not the end all! Remember Jay from the beginning of this book? As a child yoga helped him find peace; as he grew he turned to other forms of physical activity to provide nervous relief. He was able to take *yoga* with him into other disciplines that he found more engaging with age, however in times of great stress he continues to turn to *yogic breathing* to calm the nerves.

Regular practice of asana and pranayama train the body to better handle life's stressors. Asana (yoga pose) releases tight muscles with controlled movement. When looking at a particular pose there are 3 key segments, the movements into the pose, holding the pose and then the movement out of the pose. Each of these elements contributes in a positive way to the release of stress from any given muscle group. The movement into & out of a pose strengthens muscles, calms nervous energy putting it to better use and brings awareness to particular muscle groups. Holding a pose for any length of time (even just a second) allows that muscle group to lengthen, strengthen, relax and oxygenate.

Over the next few pages we will look at how to get into and out of particular poses that have a proven track record of stress management. Depending on your particular situation different asana may be of better benefit. If you wish to practice these poses on your own try to do them in order that they are written. If you are practicing alone remember that yoga is not supposed to hurt! A bit of discomfort is to be expected, especially if you are new to practice. If you feel pain back out of the pose to the point where you feel the muscles working but do not experience pain. Each day will be different. Your body changes with respect to your activities for the day or the previous day, it responds to weather, stress and a number of other stimuli. So be compassionate with yourself. You may be able to fold completely in half today with head to knees but tomorrow or next week can only come half way. It's OKAY! Listen to your body!

Keep in mind that finding a knowledgeable yoga therapist is the best way to build a personal practice that will support you in all of your physical and mental needs.

Tadasana – Standing Mountain Pose

Stand with big toes touching, heels slightly apart. Lift and spread your toes and the balls of your feet, then lay them gently back down. Rock back and forth and side to side; slowly reduces this movement to a standstill, so that your weight is balanced evenly on both feet.

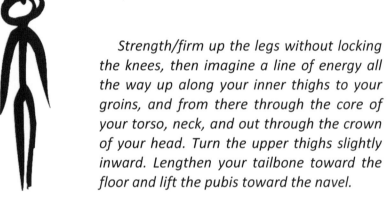

Strength/firm up the legs without locking the knees, then imagine a line of energy all the way up along your inner thighs to your groins, and from there through the core of your torso, neck, and out through the crown of your head. Turn the upper thighs slightly inward. Lengthen your tailbone toward the floor and lift the pubis toward the navel.

Press your shoulder blades into your back, then widen them across and release them down your back. Without pushing the ribs forward, lift the top of your sternum straight toward the ceiling. Widen your collarbones. Hang your arms beside the torso with palms facing front.

Balance the crown of your head directly over the center of your pelvis, with the underside of your chin parallel to the floor, throat soft, and the tongue wide and flat on the floor of your mouth. Soften your eyes.

Forward Fold

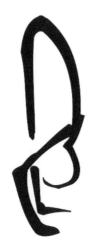

Standing Mountain inhale and lift the arms overhead without raising the shoulders, on the exhale fold forward from the hips, hands to the ground, moving the torso as one unit.

If you have long hamstrings, you can bring your forehead to your shins. If the hamstrings are short, focus on keeping the torso long. Hunching into a forward bend isn't safe for your lower back and does nothing to lengthen your hamstrings.

With each inhale allow the body to loosen and come out of the fold a little. On each exhale push a little deeper into the fold bringing the chest closer and closer to the shins. Remember to maintain length of the spine without rounding. Hold this pose for 1 to 2 minutes.

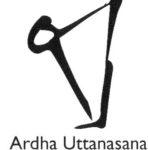

Ardha Uttanasana
Standing Half Forward Bend

On an inhale sweep the arms up with the body returning to standing Mountain Pose.

Seated Forward Fold

Sit up with legs straight out in front. Shift forward onto the sitting bones by placing your hands just behind the hips, push up so that the buttocks are raised from the ground. Now tilt the pelvis back and settle down.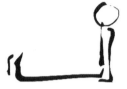

Tighten your leg muscles pushing the backs of the thighs, calves and heels into the floor; toes toward the ceiling. On an inhale raise the arms above the head lengthening the spine, keeping the shoulders down and back, keeping this length fold forward from the hips as far as you can go releasing the hands to the legs. If it is within your reach, using the index finger and thumb, grasp the big toe. Do not let the heels come off the floor.

Remember the fold comes from the hips, keeping the spine as straight as possible. With each inhale lengthening out the spine from the crown of the head down to the tailbone. With each exhale allow the fold to deepen keeping any length you gain on the inhale.

It is ok to allow the body to move slightly to the rhythm of your breath, coming up and extending on an inhale and down on an exhale.

Downward Facing Dog

Come onto your hands and knees setting the knees directly below the hips and hands slightly forward of your shoulders. Spread your palms, index fingers parallel or slightly turned out, and turn your toes under.

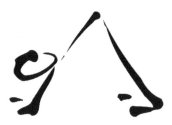

Exhale and lift your knees away from the floor. Lengthen the tailbone towards the ceiling. Inhale as you settle in, with an exhalation, push the thighs back and stretch the heels towards the floor. Straighten your knees being sure not to lock them.

Press the hands firmly into the floor actively using the entire hand. Firm the shoulder blades against your back then widen them and draw toward the tailbone. Keep the head between the upper arms; don't let it hang.

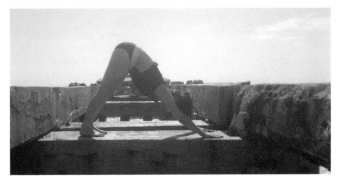

Bhujangasana - Cobra Pose

Bhujangasana otherwise known as cobra pose is said to destroy disease by increases body heat by traditional yoga texts. This pose is great for opening the heart center and relieving stress and fatigue. A great pose for asthmatics or those that experience shortness of breath as it opens the chest and makes room for the lungs to expand. The 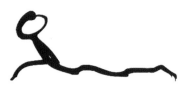 back is strengthened with this pose which helps to relieve sciatic and low back pain.

To Do:

Come onto your stomach on your mat, legs stretched long and tops of the feet on the floor.

Press the pubic bone, thighs and tops of feet into the floor.

On an inhale lift the chest away from the floor, hands firmly planted, neck long and pubis pressing into the floor. Maintain length in the spine only lifting so far as you do not feel any crunching of the vertebrae.

Hold for 3 to 5 full breaths then release back to the ground. Right cheek comes to the floor.

Take a few calming breaths and then lift once more, hold for 3 to 5 breaths.

Coming down with left ear to the floor.

Repeat once more to complete 3 lifts.

Matsyasana (Fish Pose)

This pose can be supported for a more restorative experience or done without support to fire muscles. This pose improves posture, strengthen he muscles of the upper back and neck while lengthening the muscles of the front torso. Here is another pose that is said to be combat dis-ease of the body and mind.

To do:

Lay on your back with legs either straight out or knees bent, feet flat. As you inhale lift your hips off the floor to slide your hands, palms down under the buttocks. Allow the hips to come back down resting onto your hands. Make sure the arms are close to your sides.

On an inhale bring the shoulder blades together and press your forearms into the floor. Inhale and press your forearms and elbows firmly against the floor. Lift the upper torso and head away from the floor bringing the head to rest on the coming to rest on the crown of your head or the back of the head depending on your back bend. The weight is in your arms not your head.

The knees can be bent or the legs may be long on the ground.

Hold for 3 to 5 breaths and release back to the floor on an

exhale.

To do supported:

Place 2 blocks as shown in the picture.

Lie back onto the blocks so that your head and upper back rest on the blocks.

You may remain here for up to 10 minutes, breathing deeply through your diaphragm.

Setu Bandha Sarvangasana - Bridge Pose

Bridge pose targets the lower abdominal region and helps to relieve feelings of stress. Unlike other chest opening poses bridge helps to calm the nervous system by tucking chin to chest as in a forward fold. This allows the body to benefit from the chest opener and the forward fold in one easy pose that can be done in such a way as to strengthen and lengthen muscles or supported to relax muscles.

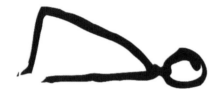

If you have suffered a neck injury do not attempt this pose on your own, seek professional advice first.

To Do:

Lie on the floor on your back, a folded blanket may be placed under the shoulders and neck for support.

Bend at the knees making sure that the ankles are directly under the knees, use an exhale to press forearms into the floor as you lift the pelvis up being sure to keep the thighs and feet parallel.

Keep lifting the pelvis up until the thighs come parallel to the floor with knees directly over heels.

The neck is long with feelings of the sternum moving towards the chin and the chin lifting away from the sternum.

Yoga is about opposing forces working together to create space and stability!

For the supported version place a yoga block or cushions under the hips and allow the body to rest onto the support. In the picture below a block is used in the highest setting for support. Play with the height, settling into the most comfortable variation for you. Remember that supported; this is a restorative pose, you should be able to stay in the position for several minutes without discomfort.

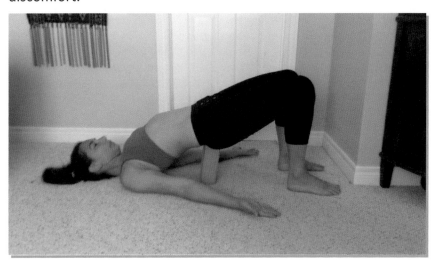

Salamba Sarvangasana - Supported Shoulder Stand

This pose helps to calm the brain, relieving stress and mild depression; it also stimulates the thyroid and prostate glands. Do not do this pose if you have a neck injury, high blood pressure or during a headache. Please note that this is an intermediate pose so if you are unsure in any way move on and seek out a teacher to guide you until you are comfortable.

To Do

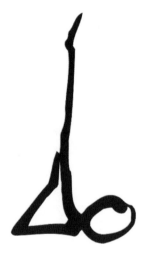

Lie on you back with shoulders supported by folded blankets or towels. Arms come to rest beside you. Curl your knees into the chest with hands pressing firmly into the floor.

Lift the back away from the floor by curling the pelvis towards the face. Brings your palms to support the back with upper arms pressing into the ground. Be mindful of the position of the upper arms along the floor, keeping them straight, in-line with the body from shoulders to hips.

Walk your hands up you back until the torso becomes perpendicular to the floor. Straighten the legs towards the ceiling. Lifting through the balls of the feet.

Keep the face and throat soft with the chin perpendicular to the floor; imagine lifting the spine away from the floor.

Hold here for 30 seconds working your way up to 3 minutes by gradually adding 5 seconds each time you practice this pose.

To come down bend the knees into the chest and roll the back slowly down to the ground. Lengthen out the body and stay resting for several minutes before getting up.

If you find this pose too intense or if you have neck problems do "legs up the wall" instead.

Viparita Karani - Legs-up-the-Wall Pose

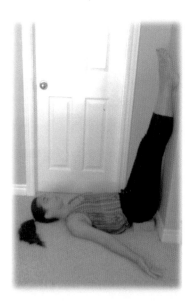

Legs up the Wall is considered a passive version of shoulder stand that is safe for everyone. Regular practice of this pose has been shown to reduce and/or completely relieve the symptoms of: Anxiety, Arthritis, Digestive problems, Headache, Insomnia, Migraine, Mild depression, Respiratory ailments, Urinary disorders, Varicose veins, Menstrual cramps, Premenstrual syndrome. Regular practice helps to regulate blood pressure.

If the feet begin to tingle bend the knees, then slide the outer edges of the feet down the wall bringing soles together with heels coming close to the pelvis.

To Do:

This pose may be supported with a block or cushion under the hips or the body resting on the ground.

Position your body perpendicular to a wall lying either supported or unsupported on your back. Use an exhale to swing your legs up the wall.

Align your body so that your "sitting" bones are close to the wall. If you feel like your neck needs support use a small rolled up towel for support. Reset the arms out to the sides, palms up.

To come out of the pose first slide out any supports you may be using. Bend your knees into your chest and roll onto the right side, stay here for a few breaths before pushing yourself up to a seated position.

Jennifer Heard

30 Minute – Short Sequence

The following script was used as a test sequence for 3 months by a small group of adults with Tourette Syndrome. They received this transcript along with a video to follow to practice at home 3 times a week. Everyone who participated fully experienced a reduction of tics over a 3 month period, with 60% tic free by the third month. Those that only practiced 1-2 times weekly still reported a reduction of tics though not as substantial. The following few pages are the transcript:

Stand with feet hip distance apart. Imagine your feet are firmly rooted to the ground; stand tall knees above ankles, hips above knees. As you inhale feel your lungs inflate, draw the ribcage in as you exhale and stack shoulders over hips, neck grows long as your chin draws parallel to the floor. As you stand in **Tadasana, Standing Mountain Pose**, feel the earth firm beneath your rooted feet. The torso feels light as the lungs fill with air.

On your next inhale slowly raise your arms wide to the sides and high above the head.

Exhale to fold forward from the hips. Take a moment and allow the legs to walk themselves out. Bending and straightening each knee to release any tension in the legs. Clasp opposite elbows as the body hangs limp over strong, rooted legs. Allow the head to sway, maybe nodding yes, shaking no, as tension falls out of the neck. Begin to slow your movements down until you find a still point.

On your next inhale lift the body half way up so that the torso is perpendicular to the legs. Bringing hands to shins or thighs to create a long straight spine. Exhale to fold keeping this new found length. Inhale sweeping the arms wide to bring them over head as you stand tall. Release the hands down through heart center as you breathe out.

Once more inhale the arms wide overhead exhale to fold inhale to rise half way, exhaling fold as you place hands on the floor allowing the knees to bend as needed. With step back with the right foot followed by the left into a plank position. Making sure that shoulders are stacked over wrists.   Paying close attention to position of the hips so that you do not sway into the spine or pike the hips. Think a long lean line from heels to head. Take a moment to breathe.

With your next exhale use the core muscles to pull the hips high to the sky with hands firmly rooted press the heels to the ground. The neck is soft as the upper arms spiral out and the shoulders move back and down the spine to create length in the neck. **Adho Mukha Svanasana, Downward Facing Dog.** Feel the pull of the hips high as the heels continue to press towards the earth. Relax into your breath allow the belly to swell and contract as you breathe life into the spine.

With your next inhale lift the right leg to the sky creating a straight line from shoulders to toes keeping length and integrity of the spine use the exhale to bring the right foot forward between the hands. Inhale to raise the body into a high lunge. As you exhale plant the left foot toes at a right angle to the right foot opening the hips and the torso arms open wide parallel to the ground looking over the right shoulder for **virabhdrasana II (warrior 2)**. Sink into your stance right thigh parallel to the ground, making sure that your knee is directly over the ankle and tracking towards the right. If your look down you should be able to see your right big toe. The left leg is strong and you feel the earth firmly through all corners of the foot. With an inhale step the left foot a bit closer to the right, inhale to straighten the right knee.

Keeping your body open to the left use the exhale bend over the right leg placing your right hand on the floor or a block as the left leg comes straight out to the side for **ardha chandrasana (half-moon pose)**. The left arm may stay on the hip or you may wish to reach for the sky. Looking towards the ground will provide the greatest stability, for a little more you can look straight ahead or for something a bit more challenging look up to the sky. Use an inhale to reach with the left hand to bring the body upright lightly placing the left foot to the ground. Sink back into warrior II.

Inhale to rotate the body forward closing the hips. The left foot comes into the ball of the foot into a high lunge. Arms rise over head. Exhale to fold from the hips placing hands firmly on the ground. Breathe. Exhale to step back into plank then inhale the hips to the sky for downdog.

Looking between your hands make your way to the top of your mat into a forward fold. Again feel the strength of the legs rooting firmly into the ground as the torso becomes light with the breath. Relax into your fold.

Inhale to come half way up, hands to shins or thighs, with a long straight spine. Exhale to fold fully keeping this length. Inhale arms wide to rise up, exhale the hands come to heart centre.

Close your eyes and feel your body. Take a quick scan as you notice any imbalances from working one side. Open your eyes as the hands release to your sides. Standing in Tadasana find your strength inhale arms over head exhale to dive forward over the legs inhale half way lift exhale to plant the hands and step back with the left foot followed by the right into plankasana.

With your next exhale pull the hips to sky with hands firmly rooted pressing heels to ground. Keeping the neck soft and the shoulders down and back. Adho mukha svanasana, downward facing dog. Feel the pull of the hips high as the heels continue to press towards the earth. Relax into your breath allow the belly to swell and contract as you breathe life into the spine.

With your next inhale raise the left leg to the sky creating a straight line from shoulders to toes keeping length of the spine use the exhale to bring the left foot forward between the hands. Inhale to raise the body into a high lunge. As you exhale plant the right foot, toes at a right angle to the left foot. Opening the hips and the torso, arms wide, parallel to the ground looking over the left shoulder for virabhdrasana II, warrior 2. Sink into your stance left thigh parallel to the ground, making sure that your knee is directly over the ankle and tracking towards the left. If your look down you should be able to see your left big toe. The right leg is strong and you feel the earth firmly through all corners of the foot. With an inhale step the right foot a bit closer to the left, right hand comes to right hip, inhale to straighten the left knee.

Keeping your body open to the right use the exhale bend and over the left leg placing your left hand on the floor or a block as the right leg comes straight out to the side for ardha chandrasana, half-moon pose. The right arm may stay on the hip or you may wish to reach for the sky. Look where you feel the most comfortable. Use an inhale to reach with the right hand to bring the body upright lightly placing the right foot to the ground. Sink back into warrior II.

Inhale to rotate the body forward closing the hips. The right foot comes onto the ball of the foot into a high lunge. Arms rise over head. Exhale to fold from the hips placing hands firmly on the ground. Breathe. Exhale to step back into plank then inhale the hips to the sky for downdog.

Looking between your hands make your way to the top of your mat into a forward fold. Once more feel the strength of your legs rooting firmly into the ground as the torso becomes light with the breath. Relax into your fold.

Place your hands firmly on the ground, the knees may bend. Exhale to push back into downdog. Inhale dropping the knees to ground, exhale to melt the chest to the floor arms extended out in front. The hips are stacked above knees, pulling high to the sky, feet flat on the floor in line with the knees. Breathe into **extended puppy; Uttana Shishosana.** With forehead on the ground breathe into the back as your spine lengthens. Release back onto your heels for **Balasana, child's Pose.** Reconnect with your breath, feel the belly expand, pressing into or between your thighs, with the inhale and contract away, pulling belly button into the spine as you exhale.

On an inhale bring the torso up to sit on your heels. Tuck the toes under, inhale to raise the arms over head, exhale hands down through heart center. Breathe into the feet.

Come forward into table top lift your feet and circle out the ankles, flex and point your toes.

Make your way onto your back, bringing your knees into your chest, rock out your spine.

Place your feet on the floor with bent knees close to your bottom so that your fingertips can graze the heels. On an inhale lift the hips, roll your shoulders back so that your arms come under you. Clasp your hands close to your heels and lift the hips a bit higher. **Setu Bandha Sarvangasana, bridge pose**. You have the option here to place a block under the hips for a supported bridge. This is a more relaxing posture. Keep knees directly over the ankles and thighs are almost parallel to the floor. Feel your tailbone pressing towards the backs of the knees.

If you are on a block remove it to the side. Release slowly back to the ground rolling the spine down with and exhale.

Bring your knees into your chest, and give yourself a hug. Create a ball with your body by bringing your forehead to your knees. Inhale to release back to the ground.

Draw your legs out long; allow the feet to fall open surrendering to gravity. The arms are by your sides palms face up. Connect to your breath.

Remain in Savasana for 5 to 10 minutes. Fully surrender to gravity, with each breath feel your body grow heavier, melting into the earth. To come out of relaxation roll onto your right side knees curl into the chest, head rests on your right arm. Take your time, when you are ready use your hands to push up to seated. Inhale arms wide and overhead exhale with a sigh hands to heart.

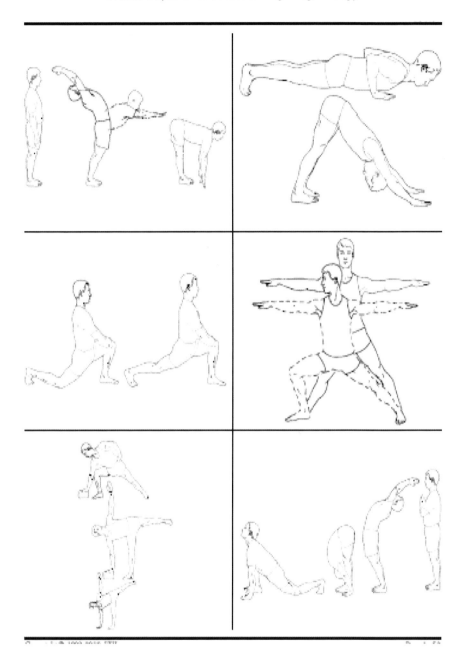

Repeat for the left side

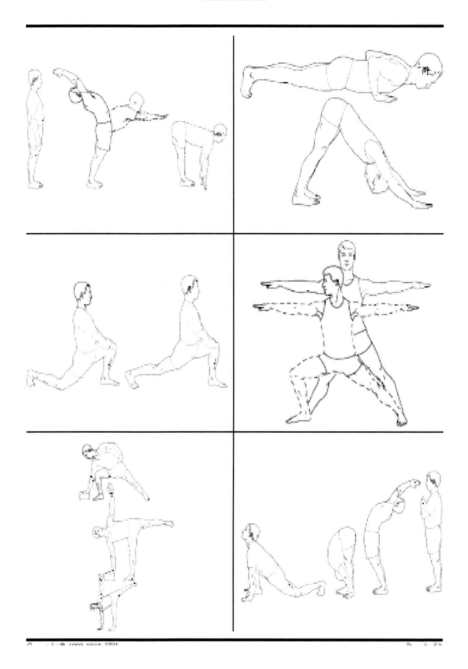

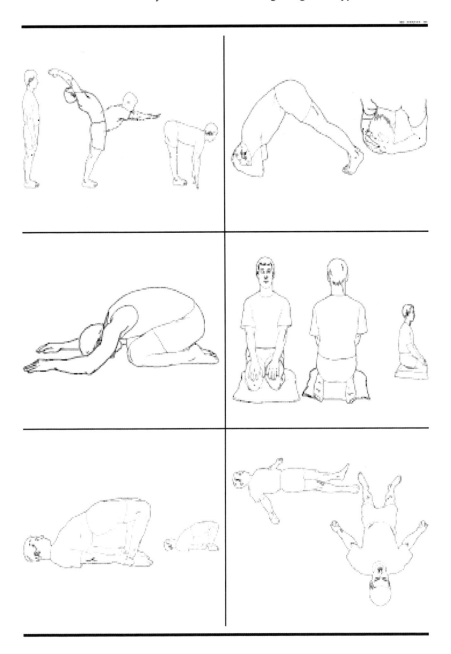

Jennifer Heard

Namaste!

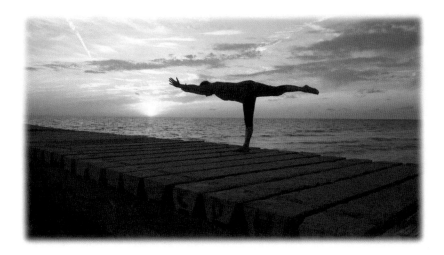

Jennifer Heard

Appendix

Jennifer Heard

Breath & Yoga Sample Journal

Date

Breath Technique

Length of Practice

Meditation

Yoga Practice

Jennifer Heard

Date:

Thoughts & Feelings Sample Journal

Use this journal format to record thoughts, feelings and the occurrence of tics as you move throughout the day.

Being mindful of your experiences without judging them. This is a very useful journal to help pinpoint physical and emotional triggers.

Morning

Mid-day

Evening

Night

Jennifer Heard

Sample Meal Journal   Date

Breakfast:
Lunch:
Supper:
Snacks:
Drinks:

Jennifer Heard

An all-encompassing journal page to let you record food, drinks exercise, thoughts and feelings in one place.

Good Eats, Bad Eats and Everything in Between!	Date
	Drinks
	Exercise
	Feelings
	Notes

Jennifer Heard

Bibliography

The neurobiology of meditation and its clinical effectiveness in psychiatric disorders; Katya Rubia, Biological Psychology. 82.1 (Sept. 2009): p1.

Differential effects of uni-nostril and alternate nostril pranayamas on cardiovascular parameters and reaction time, Ananda Bhavanani , Meena Ramanathan , R. Balaji and D. Pushpa; International Journal of Yoga. 7.1 (January-June 2014): p60

Ekman, Paul. Davidson, Richard. *The Nature of Emotion* New York. Oxford University Press 1994

Katsilambros, N. Dimosthenopoulos, C. Kontogianni, M. Manglara, E. Poulia, KA. *Clinical Nutrition in Practice*. Wiley-Blackwell Publishing 2010

Lad, Vasant. *Textbook of Ayurveda: A complete Guide to Clinical Assessment*. New Mexico. The Ayurvedic Press 2006

Myers, Thomas. *Anatomy Trains*. Elsevier Limited 2009

McCall, Timothy. *Yoga as Medicine*. New York. Bantam Books 2007

Swami Saradananda. *The Power of Breath*. London. Duncan Baird Publishers 2009

Emotional Regulation. An IAYT seminar with Rick Panico MD, 2009

Physiology of Stress and Stress Relief McCall, Timothy. SYTAR 2009

Investigating the effects of the 8-week Yoga for the Mind course on mild depression and anxiety. Ugargol, Veena C. Mason, Heather F. Gibson, Leigh. Khalsa, Sat Bir S. SYTAR 2011

The Effects of Yoga on Anxiety in Older Adults.   Bonura, Kimberlee MS, RYT. SYTAR 2008

I would to give a special thank you to Charlotte Bradley for her lovely yoga drawings! To purchase your own set of Yoga Stick Figures visit her web site:

www.yogaflavoredlife.com

ABOUT THE AUTHOR

Jennifer Heard has been studying yoga for over 15 years and natural medicine for over 10 years, earning a Doctorate of Natural Medicine with a yoga therapy specialist in the spring of 2014.

She believes that Education is the best defense and that there is a time and place for every type of medical intervention. Jennifer hopes that one day practitioners of every modality can learn to work together offering up each other's strengths to help everyone find their version of perfect health.

To learn more about or to contact Jennifer visit:

www.naturaljenn.com

www.kwyoatherapy.com

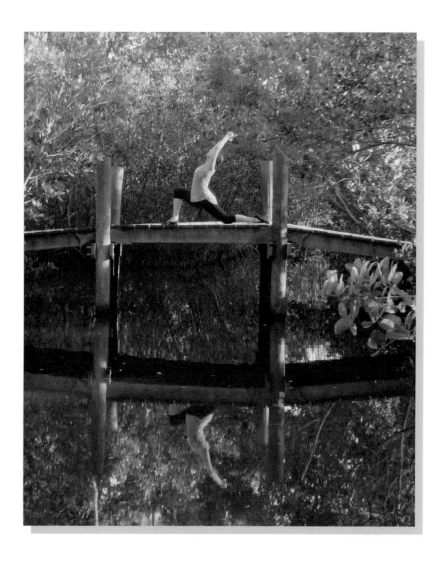

Made in the USA
Columbia, SC
30 July 2018